Health Benefits of Cranberries

For Cooking and Healing

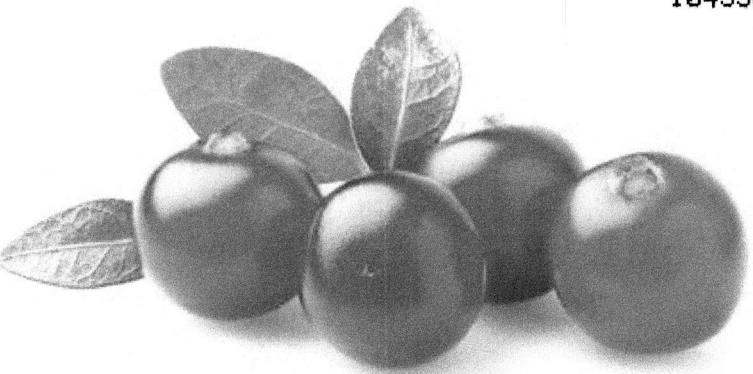

Health Learning Series
M. Usman

Mendon Cottage Books

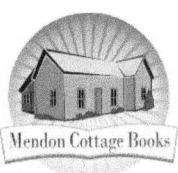

JD-Biz Publishing

All Rights Reserved.

No part of this publication may be reproduced in any form or by any means, including scanning, photocopying, or otherwise without prior written permission from JD-Biz Corp Copyright © 2014

All Images Licensed by Fotolia and 123RF.

Disclaimer

The information is this book is provided for informational purposes only. It is not intended to be used and medical advice or a substitute for proper medical treatment by a qualified health care provider. The information is believed to be accurate as presented based on research by the author.

The contents have not been evaluated by the U.S. Food and Drug Administration or any other Government or Health Organization and the contents in this book are not to be used to treat cure or prevent disease.

The author or publisher is not responsible for the use or safety of any diet, procedure or treatment mentioned in this book. The author or publisher is not responsible for errors or omissions that may exist.

Warning

The Book is for informational purposes only and before taking on any diet, treatment or medical procedure, it is recommended to consult with your primary health care provider.

Our books are available at

1. Amazon.com
2. Barnes and Noble
3. Itunes
4. Kobo
5. Smashwords
6. Google Play Books

Table of Contents

Getting Started

Chapter # 1: Intro

Cranberries are one of the most popular berries around the globe and are well-known for their delicious use in holiday celebrations; in the form of drinks, sauces and stuffing. What most people don't know, are the vast, and largely ignored, health benefits of this berry. Wild, unique and natural by habitat, cranberries are rich in health-promoting materials that are essential for all year wellness. And that's not all; cranberries are known to store agents that protect against ailments like cancer and cardiovascular threats. But, before jumping into the health benefits, it is essential that you have a good understanding of the berry itself, so read on and learn.

For starters, it should be known that cranberries are part of the same family as that of blueberries: *Vaccinium*. Scarlet red, glossy and tart in appearance, cranberries are evergreen shrubs that may be classified as trailing vines, growing to very low heights of usually 10-20 cm and a length of 2 meters. They are also called "bounce berries" by some because of their ability to bounce upon reaching ripeness. The name cranberry is thought to be derived from the fact that their pink blossoms are visually similar to the heads of cranes that are bogged by cranberries. Cranberries can be found in most of the northern hemisphere and are characterized by slender, wiry stems, which are not at all woody, and have evergreen leaves. The fruit of the shrub is a berry that is larger in size when compared to the leaves, of white color initially, turns deep red on reaching ripeness and of acidic taste that largely overpowers its sweetness. Cranberries contain the highest load of beneficial nutrients at their peak, i.e. during the months of October and December. This time period coincides with major holidays like Thanksgiving, making cranberries an integral part of holiday meals.

It is a recorded fact that American Indians used cranberries extensively in their everyday life, enjoying them in both cooked & sweetened form along with maple syrup & honey. Furthermore, they used it as a decoration, a source of red dye and for medicinal properties that included healing wounds and stopping bleeding. In the Colonial World, cranberry sauce was considered a treat at Thanksgiving feasts and before long these berries were being exported to England by the colonists. Even though many cranberries species were and are found in parts of Asia and Europe, the American derivative proved to be the most cultivated and preferred one. It owes its success to a common yet observant gentleman named Henry Hall.

In 1840, Henry noticed that due to prevailing winds & tides, sand had swept in his bog and as a result an abundance of cranberries had grown in that area. It was found that the sandy bog gave just the correct conditions for cranberries to stifle their shallow-rooted weeds and enhanced the growth of deep rooted ones.

Soon cranberry cultivation spread not only across the US, through the states of Wisconsin to Washington & Oregon but also across the Atlantic to Scandinavian countries and Britain. The berries made their way into Holland the hard way; when a US ship loaded with crates packed with cranberries sank along the Dutch coast. Some of the berries sank ashore on the island of Tershelling and took root there, making their way into the Dutch population. As stated earlier, because American variation of the cranberries is preferred, the Northern American continent is the major supplier of the world's cranberries. In the Canadian state of British Colombia alone, 20% of the world's cranberries are harvested. Other countries with small yet significant productions include Chile, Argentina, Netherlands and the Eastern European region.

But along with being a festive treat, there is also a health promoting side of cranberries. Cranberries are one of the healthiest foods and are often at the top of nutrition lists for their high antioxidant content. Not to mention, a half cup of cranberries are filled with only 25 calories which makes it an excellent food for people with strict diet plans.

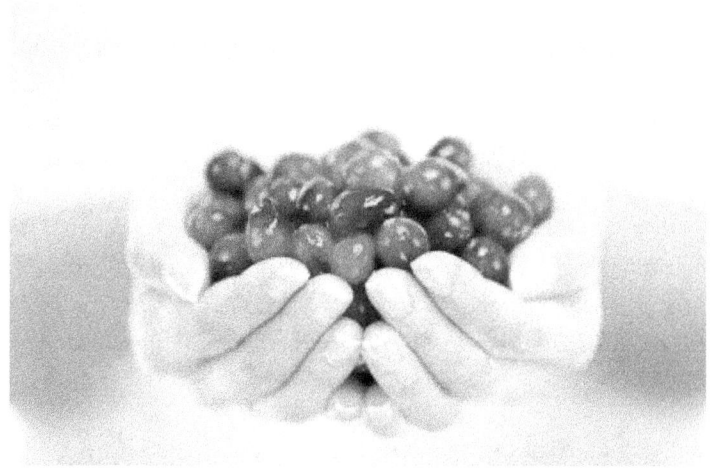

The major health-promoting effects of cranberries include:

- These delicious, tart berries have noticeably high amounts of extremely nutritious compounds called phytochemicals that fight against aging, cancer, neurological diseases, diabetes, inflammation and infections.

- Cranberries are also rich in antioxidant compounds that buck up the cardiovascular system by countering against cholesterol plaque build-up in blood vessels and heart. Plus, these compounds lower the levels of bad cholesterol in the body while raising the level of the good one.

- Cranberry juice can protect against bacterial infections in the urinary system. It also helps to prevent urinary stones by battling against a different type of bacterial infection.

- They prevent plaque formation on the surface of the teeth.

- They are a great source of nutrients like vitamin C, A, B and minerals like potassium & manganese which hold countless benefits on their own.

Detailed analysis of the health benefits as well as nutrient composition is provided in the following chapters. Follow the book, chapter by chapter and you'll soon find out all the good stuff you've been missing.

Chapter # 2: Nutritional Worth

Along with being an important and traditional holiday feast, cranberries are packed with an array of nutrients and minerals. They contain the infamous vitamin C and are therefore very effective antioxidants. In fact, cranberries beat almost every fruit in antioxidant content including heavy weight contenders like spinach, broccoli, strawberries, red grapes, raspberries, apples and cherries. Statistically speaking, a cup of cranberries has a total of 8,983 antioxidant capacities; this number is toppled by only the blueberry and no other.

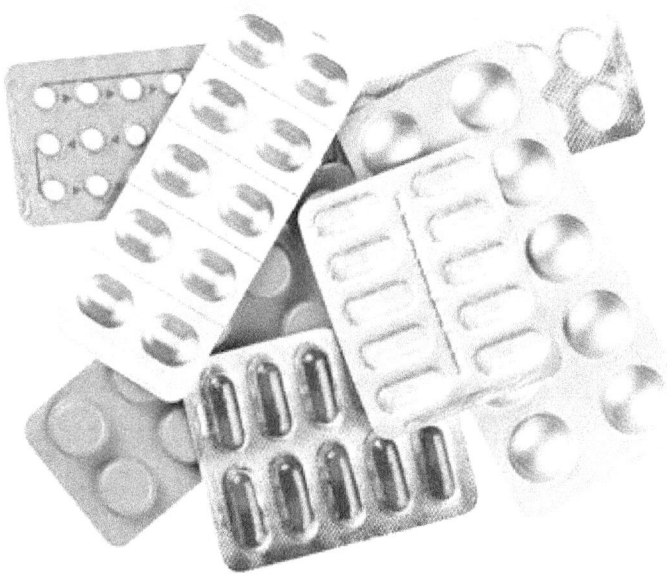

Many times, the power of vitamin C is undermined by many so it must be clarified that this particular vitamin is a very strong natural antioxidant that is capable of blocking most if not all damage that is a result of free radicals. Along with this, vitamin C can also protect the body against infectious diseases. During older times, sailors tended to carry cranberries with them to avoid scurry, a disease caused by lack of vitamin C. Another very influential vitamin, vitamin E is present in cranberries that boost the immune system and helps prevent chronic diseases.

Fiber is another nutritious element of cranberries which, according to the Department of Internal Medicine and Nutritional Sciences, results in lowering the risk of cardiovascular diseases like stroke, hypertension, diabetes, obesity and coronary heart disease. Fiber is also known for its property to lower blood pressure, cholesterol levels and improving insulin sensitivity that is directly linked to weight loss.

Cranberries also contain manganese, vitamin K, and a wide variety of phytonutrients that occur in plant chemicals and help prevent countless ailments and diseases. The health benefits of each of these along with previously mentioned nutrients have been discussed in the forthcoming section.

A detailed account of the nutritional wellness of cranberries is given in the following table. The amount taken is 100 grams.

Calorie Information	
Nutrient	Amount
Total Calories	46.0
From Carbohydrates	43.6
From Fat	1.1
From Proteins	1.3
Carbohydrates	
Nutrient	Amount
Total Carbohydrates	12.2 g
Dietary Fiber	4.6 g
Starch	0.0 g

Sugar	4.0 g

Fats & Fatty Acids

Nutrient	Amount
Total Fat	0.1 g
Saturated Fat	0.0 g
Mono-saturated Fat	0.0 g
Polyunsaturated Fat	0.1 g
Total Omega-3 Fatty acids	22.0 mg
Total Omega-6 Fatty acids	33.0 mg

Proteins

Nutrient	Amount
Protein	0.4 g

Vitamins

Nutrient	Amount
Vitamin A	60 IU
Vitamin C	13.3 mg
Vitamin E	1.2 mg
Vitamin K	5.1 mcg
Thiamin	0.0 mg
Riboflavin	0.0 mg

Niacin	0.1 mg
Vitamin B6	0.1 mg
Folate	1.0 mcg
Vitamin B12	0.0 mg
Pantothenic Acid	0.3 mg
Choline	5.5 mg

Minerals

Nutrient	Amount
Calcium	8.0 mg
Iron	0.3 mg
Magnesium	6.0 mg
Phosphorus	13.0 mg
Potassium	85.0 mg
Sodium	2.0 mg
Zinc	0.1 mg
Copper	0.1 mg
Manganese	0.4 mg
Selenium	0.1 mcg

Chapter # 3: Selection and Storage

Cranberry is a fruit with a relatively short season; fresh cranberries are harvested at their peak between Labor Day and Halloween and begin to appear in markets throughout the months of October through December. When buying from a store or fruit shop, be sure to choose fresh, deep red in color, firm to the touch and plump cranberries. Discard any mottled, wet berries as they tend to accumulate molds. Remember, the deeper red their color is, the more concentrated the berries' beneficial anthocyanin compounds are. Along with redness, firmness is the main indicator of a cranberry's quality; truly fresh cranberries are quite firm to the touch and bounce when dropped. During harvesting, high quality cranberries are separated from low quality ones by bouncing them against barriers composed of slanted boards. The best quality berries bounce over the barrier while the minor ones automatically collect in a separate pile. Fresh cranberries are usually available in 12 ounce plastic bags and sometimes in pint containers. Other forms of berries that are also available include dried, frozen and canned, which is a sauce of smooth texture.

Fresh ripe cranberries can be easily, and without hesitation, stored in a refrigerator for up to 20 days. There is, however, a few things you should consider before storing fresh cranberries: before storing be sure to discard any discolored, soft, pitted or shriveled berries as it can easily become breeding grounds for molds. Also, moistness of cranberries when they are taken out of the refrigerator does not indicate spoilage, unless the cranberries have a sticky, leathery or tough feel to them along with discoloration. Once frozen, the cranberries can be kept for several years but to freeze them there is also a specific procedure: first, spread the fresh cranberries on a cookie sheet and place the sheet in the freezer. After a couple of hours, the frozen berries will be ready to be transferred into a freezer bag and stored safely. (Don't forget to place the current date on the bag, just as a reminder)

Cooked cranberries can also be stored in a covered container in a refrigerator and can last up to a single month. If liquor is added to the mixture, they can last for a whole year.

While not as sensitive as blueberries, fresh cranberries still need to be treated with care and fragility. Prior to use, place the cranberries in a strainer and gently rinse them under cool, flowing water. Frozen berries that do not require cooking must be thawed well and subsequently drained before being used. For cooked recipes, the berries must be used in unthawed form as this will ensure maximum flavor.

With a health point of view, it must be stated that cranberries retain their maximum nutrients along with their taste when enjoyed fresh and not in any cooked recipe. The reason behind this is simple. Enzymes, vitamins and antioxidants are natural compounds, they are unable to withstand temperatures above 175 degrees and that's why fresh cranberries taste better when consumed in their natural form.

Chapter # 5: Individual Concerns

Cranberries are one of the few food items that contain reckonable amounts of oxalates; naturally occurring substances found in animals, humans and plants. Oxalates have been related to formation of kidney stones as these stones have been found to contain traces of oxalate compounds. In the case of cranberries, the oxalate content is quite low, 5-7 mg per 3.5 ounce, but still cranberries are able to increase the amount of oxalates as well as calcium in the urine, resulting in increased concentrations of calcium oxalate. Thereby, it is advised to individuals who are at risk of calcium oxalate kidney stone formation to avoid cranberries; if they still want to make it a part of their diets they should consult a health specialist beforehand. It should be noted that cranberries do help with preventing kidney stones including struvite stones & brushite stones but if you don't know the type of stones you have, it is best to consult a health specialist.

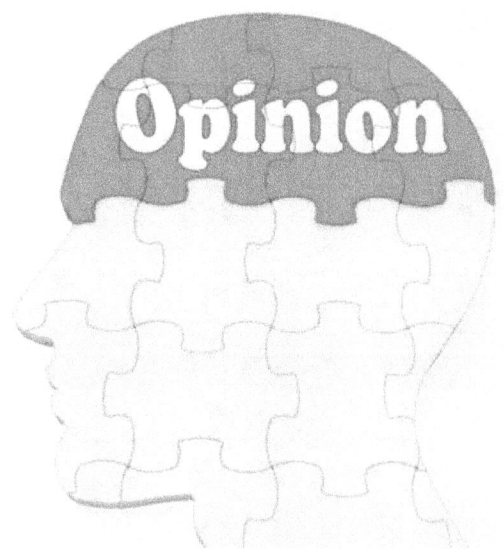

Health Benefits

Chapter # 1: Anti-Inflammatory Agent

What are phytonutrients? In extremely simple words, phytonutrients are chemicals found in plants that are beneficial to the well-being of the human body. These nutrients protect against a wide array of threats including germs, bugs, fungi and other micro-organisms. For the cardiovascular system, along with parts of the digestive tract, cranberry has shown promising anti-inflammatory effects. Phytonutrients present in cranberries namely include, proanthocyanidins (PACs), anthocyanins (the characteristic red color of cranberries), flavonols like quercitin and the infamous phenolic acid, all of which contribute to lowering the risk of inflammations.

With respect to our gums, the anti-inflammatory characteristics of cranberries help lower the risk of periodontal diseases. Excessive and chronic levels of inflammation in the region around the gums pose a threat to and damage the tissues supporting our teeth. This particular inflammation is triggered by continuous overproduction of certain chemicals known as cytokines. Cytokines are pro-inflammatory, messenger molecules responsible for launching inflammatory actions in body's cells. As these actions continue the inflammations increase and therefore cause damage to the body. Phytonutrients in cranberries combat against this inflammatory cascade right at the cytokine level. In addition, phytonutrients in cranberries inhibit the activity of chemicals that cause the production of other anti-inflammatory molecules, thereby inhibiting damage by inflammation.

Specific benefits like cardiovascular and digestive ones are discussed in greater detail in the following chapters.

Chapter # 2: Protection against Urinary & Digestive Tract Infections

Urinary tract is the scheme by which urine is carried out of the body; it includes the bladder, kidney, and tubes connecting them. When germs or micro-organisms get into this system, they cause infections known as Urinary Tract Infections. More than 150 million cases of these infections surface globally each year, with antibiotic treatment being the standard treatment for these infections. Researchers have found that there has been a rise in bacterial resistance to antibiotic treatments and therefore, a more effective way is required.

A study presented at the Experimental Biology Conference held all the way back in 2002 showed evidence that cranberries contained compounds that had the ability to protect against urinary tract infections. Amy Howell, who was a research scientist at the Mariucci Center for Blueberry-cranberry Research at Rutgers University, along with her colleague Jess Reed, carried out a study that explained why cranberry was able to provide this benefit. An eight-ounce serving of cranberry juice was served to six volunteers; it was found that the cranberry juice was able to prevent the bacteria, E. coli from sticking to bladder cells, hence protecting against UTIs. After this research, many other studies found their way into discovering the benefits of cranberries against UTIs.

Currently, treatment of Urinary Tract Infections is one of the leading areas of research when it comes to health benefits of cranberries. In fact, cranberry was in use for UTI treatments long before researchers started to investigate cranberries' properties. At one time, cranberries' acidity was considered of great importance, but soon it was found out that cranberries' ability to deliver UTI benefits was linked to its proanthocyanidin (PAC) content and not its acidity. The PACs in cranberries are special compounds with a unique structure that make it unfavorable for bacteria to latch on to the urinary tract. The bacteria that latch on to the urinary tract include the infection causing E. coli which is one of the most wide spread micro-organisms when it comes to causing UTIs. Thus, by making it hard for unwanted bacteria like the E. coli to stick onto the urinary tract, the PACs prevent the expansion of bacterial populations that ultimately end up in infections. Cranberries have shown quite pronounced benefits in middle-aged women who have experienced recurring episodes of UTIs; some studies have even shown the number to reduce by 1/3rd with dietary consumption of cranberries. However, researchers are still unsure of the benefits reaped by children and don't know if they are the same as that of middle aged people.

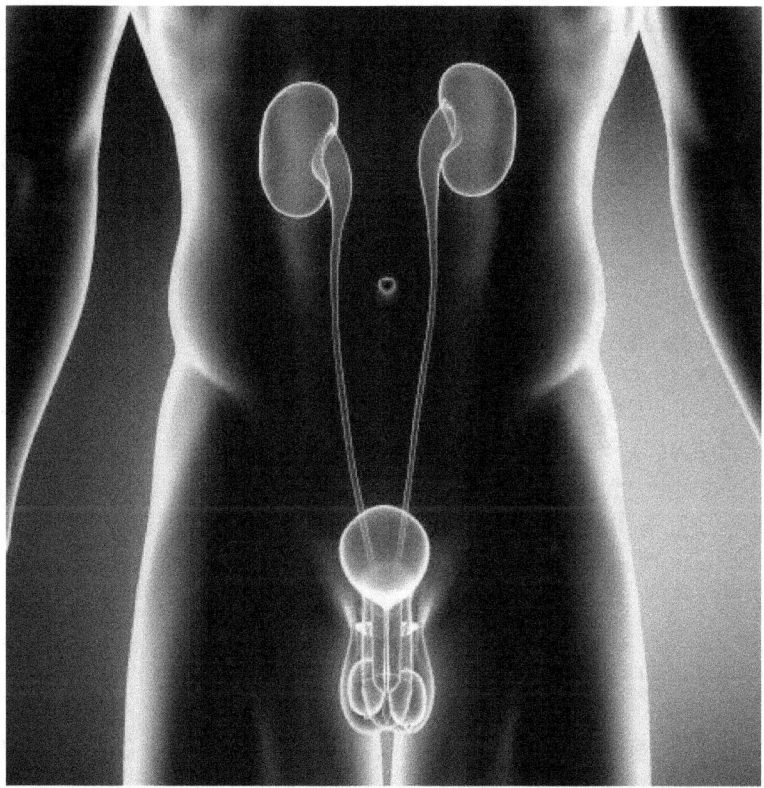

Two studies published in the Canadian Journal of Microbiology & Colloids & Surfaces have shown that cranberry powder inhibited bacteria that were the common cause of complicated urinary tract infections. Earlier studies from the same group had concluded that cranberry materials had the ability to limit the movement of micro-organisms, mainly bacteria in the urinary tracts. The research was carried out by chemical engineering scientists at Montreal's McGill University and showed that exposure to cranberry extracts decreased the density of infections. The new research showed that when the concentration of cranberry powder was increased, the bacteria's production of an enzyme that helped to spread infections, decreased. The researchers acclaimed their work as significant, stating that the movement of bacteria is the main mechanism by which bacterial infections spread; by stopping them from moving so easily, UTIs infections were decreased.

The adhesive blocking mechanism by which cranberries prevent bacteria from latching onto the urinary tract has allowed research on cranberries to expand and go beyond just UTIs and into the field of the digestive system. Almost every fruit is known to provide benefits to the digestive tract and the case is the same with cranberries. Every phytochemical found in cranberries is known to play a role in digestive health; the proanthocyanidin phytochemical lowers the occurrence of the bacterium, Helicobacter pylori whereas the flavonoids provides anti-inflammatory benefits that result in decreased risk of colon infections. One research was able to show that cranberries normalize the balance of bacteria in the digestive tract. Participants in the study were given 2 ounces of cranberry juice a day for a time period of 3 months. It was found that cranberries didn't interfere with the number of Bifidobacteria bacteria that are good for the tract; rather they decreased the number of disease causing bacterium and with that actually helped promote digestive tract health.

Chapter # 3: Prevention against Kidney Stone Formation

Kidney stones are hard masses formed in the kidneys consisting of insoluble compounds usually containing calcium. They are a result of accumulation of dissolved minerals in the inner lining of the kidneys. These deposits can keep on increasing and grow to the size of golf balls if not treated! Furthermore, they retain their sharp, crystalline structure that leads to penetrating pains in the lower body, among other displeasures.

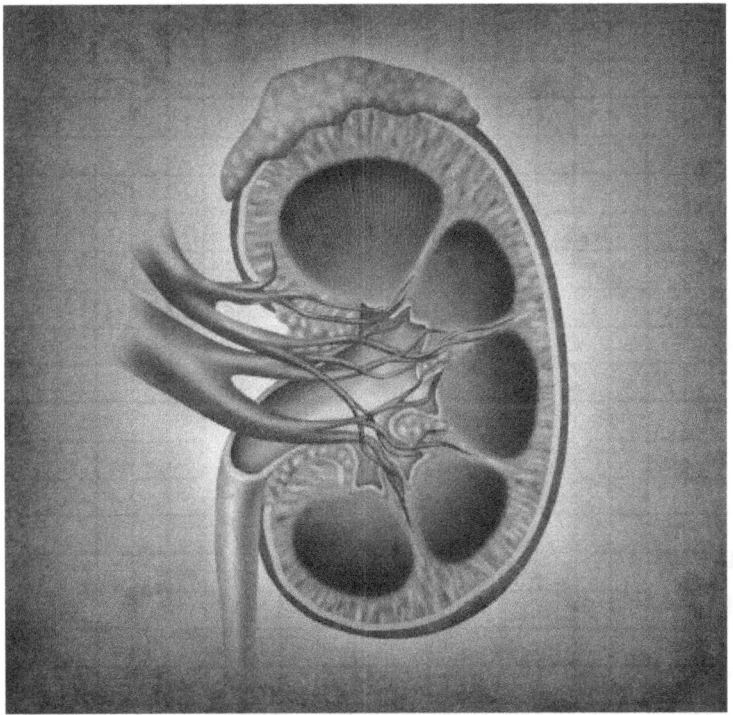

Kidney stones can be formed from several different mineral combinations, and the most common of which are the combination of calcium & oxalic acid. This combination is known as calcium-oxalate stones and is responsible for most of the cases of kidney stones in US. Other cases are due to mineral combinations of:

- Calcium & phosphate called brushite stones.

- Magnesium & sulfate called struvite stones.

- Uric acid forming urate stones.

Since cranberries are known for their ability to increase the concentration of oxalate and calcium in the urine, they can increase the likelihood of stone formation but with other mineral combinations, cranberries are actually helpful in countering the mineral buildup. For instance, urinary uric acid is a mineral combination which is decreased by the intake of cranberry, thereby decreasing the risk of urate stones formation. The bottom line is that if you do have kidney stones, its best to talk to a health professional first for incorporating cranberries in your diet. If he/she gives a green light, enjoy nature's sparkling berry with full zest.

Chapter # 4: Antioxidant & Anticancer Effect

In very simple words, antioxidants are compounds that prevent cell damage by countering free radical reactions in the body. Antioxidants found in cranberries are of special importance and contribute greatly to the well-being of the body. They are the body's first line of defense against free radicals and damage induced by them which includes risk of diseases like strokes, diabetes, arthritis, cancer and many cognitive disabilities.

Cranberries are among some of the finest fruits that are most investigated by scientists for their anti-oxidative behavior. In several separate studies, it was shown that cranberries were among the best natural food items in the fight against cancer, inhibiting common pathogens and aiding in UTIs. One study presented at the Experimental Biology's 2002 meeting showed that cranberry juice had the greatest total phenol content along with having the highest free radical scavenging ability among the fruits studied.

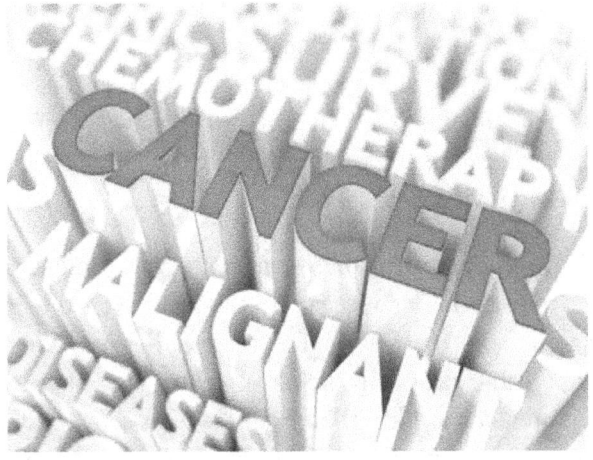

Strictly speaking from a research point of view, there are two very important things that must be considered when talking about cranberries' antioxidant benefits.

- First is the fantastic array of antioxidants, available exclusively to whole cranberries. Cranberries' unique combination of anthocyanin, proanthocyanidin, phenolic, flavonoid and triterpenoid antioxidants deliver an antioxidant pay load that combats free radicals unlike most other food items with antioxidants.

- Second is the importance of these health-promoting nutrients to be delivered in combination with each other. The array of antioxidants found in cranberries is not the real reason why cranberries prove to be so effective against free radicals; the real secret is their combination, which provides maximal health benefits to the body.

In one study carried out by an assistant professor at the University of Massachusetts-Dartmouth, several bioactive compounds from whole cranberries were extracted and studied; many of these compounds showed strong antioxidant activity and proved to be toxic against tumor cells found in lungs, prostate, breast and bone marrow.

Another thing that must be stated is that in many researches on cranberries' antioxidant properties, and it was found that cranberries were unable to deliver significant amount of antioxidant benefits. When a closer look was taken at these activities, it was found that the cranberries were at work but the results were not visible at blood level. At cellular level is was discovered and ultimately concluded those cranberries' antioxidants worked by triggering metabolic events; this gave cranberries a much stronger track record than it was previously assumed.

For the past 10 years the relation between cranberries and cancer has proven very intriguing to scientists and researchers which have led to extensive research being done on the topic. Much of the studies have been limited to lab studies on human cancer cells but nevertheless, they have established cranberries' compounds as a contributor to the fight against cancer. Researchers started out with 50,000 human cells infected with prostate cancer in an experimental dish and observed it for a few days. In a day the cells multiplied to 100,000, then 200,000 and after 3 days they reached a whopping 400,000. Now, researchers added just a tiny amount of cranberries in to the dish and observed that the exponential growth was blocked.

A very commonly diagnosed cancer is breast cancer. Epidemiological studies have continuously suggested a decrease in cancer risk by the intake of fruits & vegetables; one of these fruits is cranberries. Cranberries are known to have compounds that carry out a preemptive strike on cancer-causing mechanisms, such as halting the growth of cancer cell lines and inhibition of enzymes that lead to tumors. Researchers at the Department of Food Science at the Cornell University found out that extracts from cranberries were able to inhibit the proliferation of human breast cells when injected at doses ranging from 5-30 units (mg/mL). Cell death in these cancerous tumors was directly dependent to the amount of dose and exposure to the phytochemicals. Doses worth 50 units resulted in a 25% higher kill ratio when compared to groups without any exposure. After 24 hours the number of cancerous cells in the control group was found to be 6 times more than the exposed group effectively proving cranberries' ability to halt cancerous cells from multiplying.

Chapter # 5: Boosting the Cardiovascular System

The cardiovascular system is a complex mechanism in the human body which is entrusted with the tasks of transporting nutrients and removing gaseous waste from the body. The system comprises of the heart as its center and the circulatory system which acts as a pathway from one organ to another. The cardiovascular system is absolutely necessary for life and the whole concept of a functioning human body would collapse if this system were to face a severe damage.

It was mentioned earlier that treatment of urinary tract infections with cranberries had stirred a large number of researches on the topic and it should be noted that after urinary tract infections, the cardiovascular system is the best researched area when it comes to cranberries' benefits. The major players in promoting health in the cardiovascular system are the antioxidants and anti-inflammatory nutrients found in cranberries.

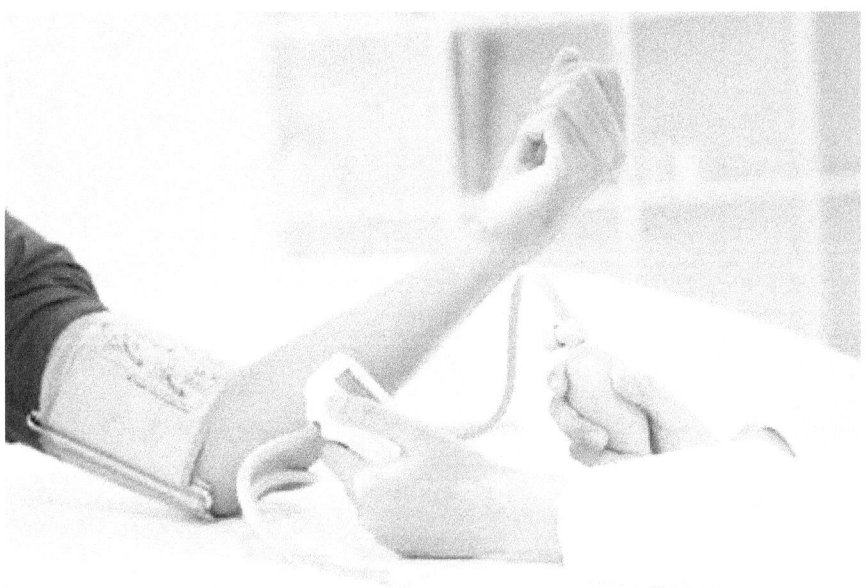

Oxidative stress along with chronic inflammation can place the walls of our blood vessels at great danger. Once damaged, the walls of the same blood vessels go under a process of plaque formation that increases the risk of atherosclerosis. Atherosclerosis is a disease that is highlighted by fatty deposits in the inner walls of arteries. Dietary intake of cranberries along with its juice has shown to prevent two enzymes from triggering which is the pivotal point in the whole process of atherosclerosis.

The antioxidants present in cranberries also have a key role in alleviating threats to the cardiovascular system. Several animal studies have shown that the intake of cranberries had a direct effect on the value of blood pressure. Cranberry extracts were responsible for reducing oxidative stress inside the blood vessels which directly caused prevention in the over constriction of blood vessels.

The final ground for cranberries, where they can provide cardiovascular support, is the ability to lower LDL cholesterol. It should be known that there are two types of cholesterol present in our bodies: one is LDL cholesterol, bad for health while the other is HDL cholesterol, good for health. Cranberries were not only able to decrease the level of LDL cholesterol but were also able to simultaneously increase the levels of HDL cholesterol. Cranberries help the body achieve these cholesterol improving modifications by improving the inflammatory & oxidative aspects of everyday environment in which cholesterol-containing compounds exist. This resulted in improved cholesterol control by normalizing the levels of HDL and LDL cholesterol that contributes to decreasing the risk of blood vessel getting blocked & problems associated with that risk.

Recipes

Chapter # 1: Cranberry Eggnog Cornbread Scones

Makes: 8 servings

Prep time: 20 minutes

Cooking time: 50 minutes

Ingredients:

- 2 cups flour, all-purpose
- 1/3 cup white sugar
- ½ cup cornmeal
- 1 tablespoon baking powder
- ½ teaspoon salt
- ¾ cup sweetened, dried cranberries
- 1/3 cup chilled butter
- 2/3 cup eggnog

Directions:

First of all, preheat the oven to 190 degrees Celsius and grease a baking sheet. Stir the cornmeal, flour, baking powder, sugar, and salt in a mixing bowl until finely blended. Take a pastry cutter and cut the butter into crumbs, and add the crumbs to the mixture prepared earlier. Toss in the cranberries and use a fork to incorporate the eggnog to make sticky dough. Extract the dough onto a floured surface and dip your hands in a little flour and knead the dough about 10 times. Pat the dough onto a ½ inch thick disk and cut out about 10 rounds of the dough using a 2 inch diameter biscuit cutter dipped in flour. As the rounds are cut, place them onto the baking sheet prepared at the start and after all the rounds have been placed, bake them in the preheated oven until they turn golden brown. Finally serve the scones warm or as per liking.

Chapter # 2: Cranberry Walnut Bread

Makes: 3 loaves

Prep time: 40 minutes

Cooking time: 1 hour

Ready in: 1 hour 40 minutes

Ingredients:

- ¾ cup butter

- 3 eggs

- 3 cups white sugar

- 3 tablespoons orange zest

- 1 tablespoon salt

- 6 cups all-purpose flour

- 4 ½ teaspoons baking powder

- 2 ¼ cups orange juice

- 1 ½ teaspoons baking soda

- 1 ½ cups chopped walnuts

- 3 cups whole cranberries

Directions:

Preheat an oven to 175 degrees Celsius and grease three 8x4 loaf pans. (If you want, use parchment paper to line the bottoms) Next, beat the sugar and butter, with the help of an electric mixer, in a large bowl until the mixture turns fluffy. Add each of the eggs, allowing each egg to blend into the mixture before the next one is added. Add the orange zest and stir it too. Sift the salt, flour, baking soda and baking powder and add it to the mixture with alternating additions of orange juice. Pour the flour mixture into a mixing bowl and add in coarsely chopped cranberries along with walnuts, mixing them so they evenly combine. Divide the batters evenly among the pans prepared in the start and bake them in the oven for 30 minutes; cover the tops with aluminum foil and bake until a fork inserted in to the middle of the loaf comes out clean. Finally cool on wire racks and serve.

Chapter # 3: Holiday Cranberry Sauce

Makes: 16 servings

Prep time: 5 minutes

Cooking time: 15 minutes

Ready in: 8 hours 20 minutes

Ingredients:

- 4 cups fresh cranberries

- 5 whole cloves

- 1 ½ cups water

- 5 whole allspice berries

- 2 cups white sugar

- 3 cinnamon sticks

Directions:

Put a sauce pan over medium heat and toss in the cranberries and water. Wrap the cloves, cinnamon sticks and berries in a spice bag and place the bag in the water being heated. Cook for 10 minutes after which you should reduce the heat to low and stir in the sugar. Continue cooking at low heat for 5 minutes or until the sugar has dissolved. Finally remove from the heat, discard the spice bag and chill in the refrigerator overnight before serving.

Conclusion

Cranberries have shown a lot of potential in major disease blocking areas and are therefore becoming the interest of several researchers. Many studies have already shown that cranberries' compounds have the ability to protect against the risk of diseases like cancer, UTIs and heart-related ones. This energetic, little berry packs a pay load of antioxidants unlike any other and, through that, is able to prevent many diseases that would otherwise turn big if left untreated. This book provides a comprehensive guide on the use of cranberries, from its literature to its recipes; not a stone has been left unturned to bring you closer to the charismatic tart that cranberry is.

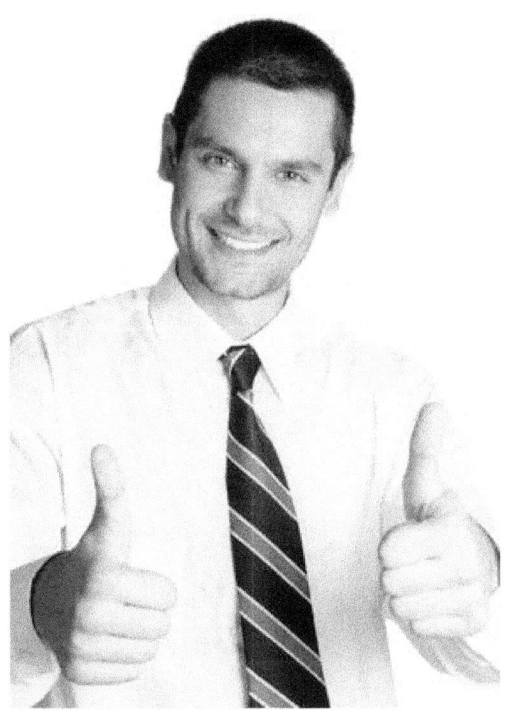

References

http://nl.123rf.com/photo_10395437_mannelijke-anatomie-van-menselijke-urogenitale-landstreek-in-x-ray-weergave.html

http://nl.123rf.com/photo_13838366_menselijke-nier-op-een-grunge-textuur-als-een-medische-diagram-met-een-doorsnede-van-de-binnenste-or.html

http://nl.123rf.com/photo_16970476_cranberry-met-bladeren-in-close-up.html

http://nl.123rf.com/photo_14943199_cranberries-vrouw-met-veenbessen-gezond-eten-en-bessen-concept-van.html

http://www.fotolia.com/id/37121015

http://www.fotolia.com/id/47533987

http://www.fotolia.com/id/49549245

http://www.fotolia.com/id/47136007

http://www.fotolia.com/id/51102457

Author Bio

Muhammad Usman is a distinguished medical graduate of Allama iqbal medical college (AIMC). He is a professional writer who has been in the field for more than 4 years. During this time he has produced 10,000+ articles, blogs and eBooks on various niches related to diseases, health, fitness, nutrition and well-being. He is a regular contributor to several journals related to medicine and surgery. He is the editor of several journals and newspapers.

Check out some of the other JD-Biz Publishing books

Gardening Series on Amazon

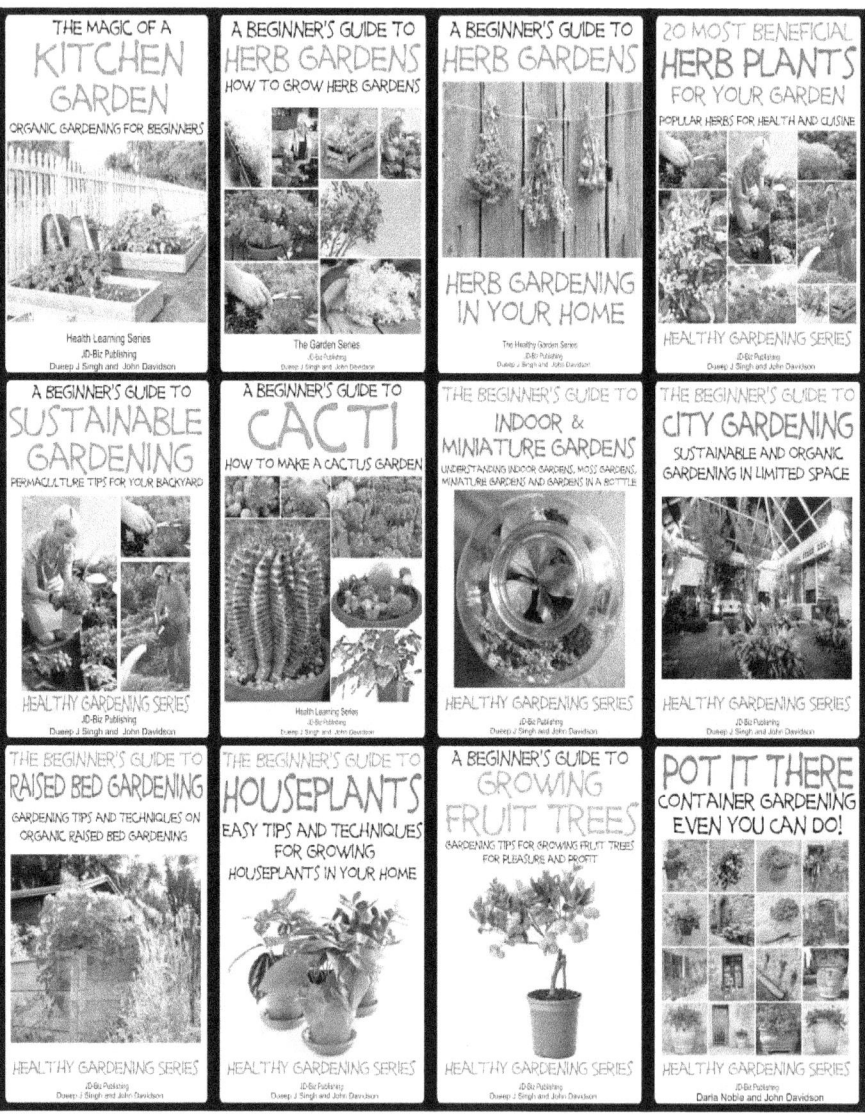

Health Learning Series

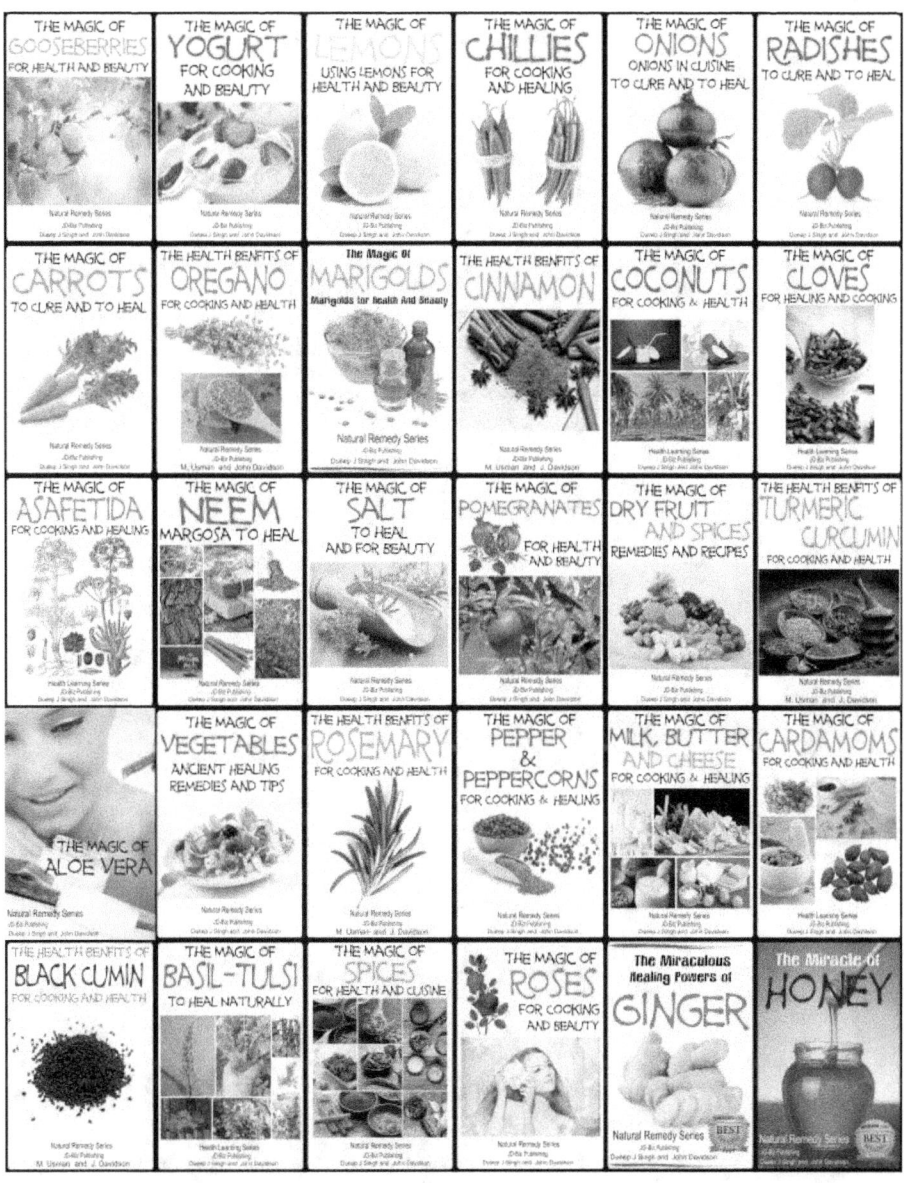

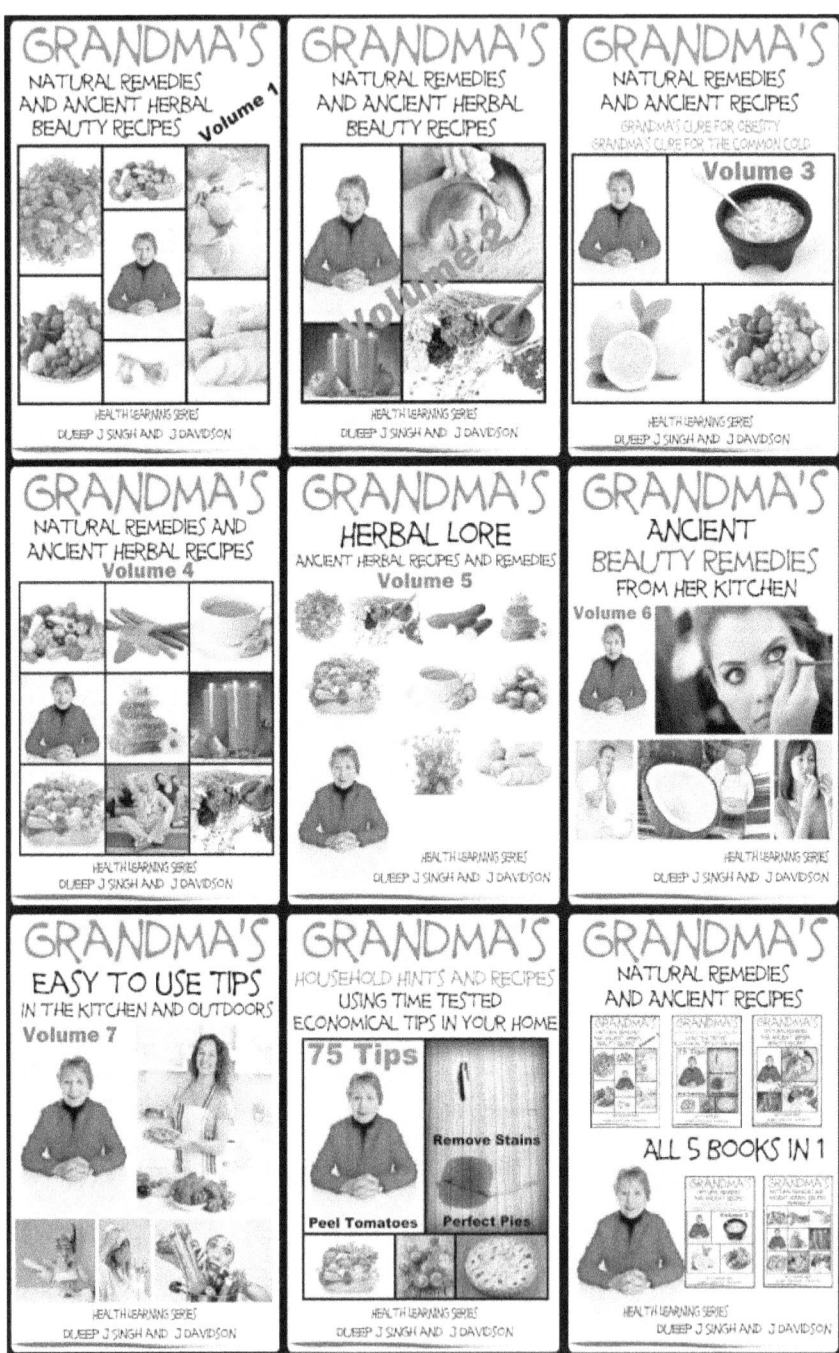

Country Life Books

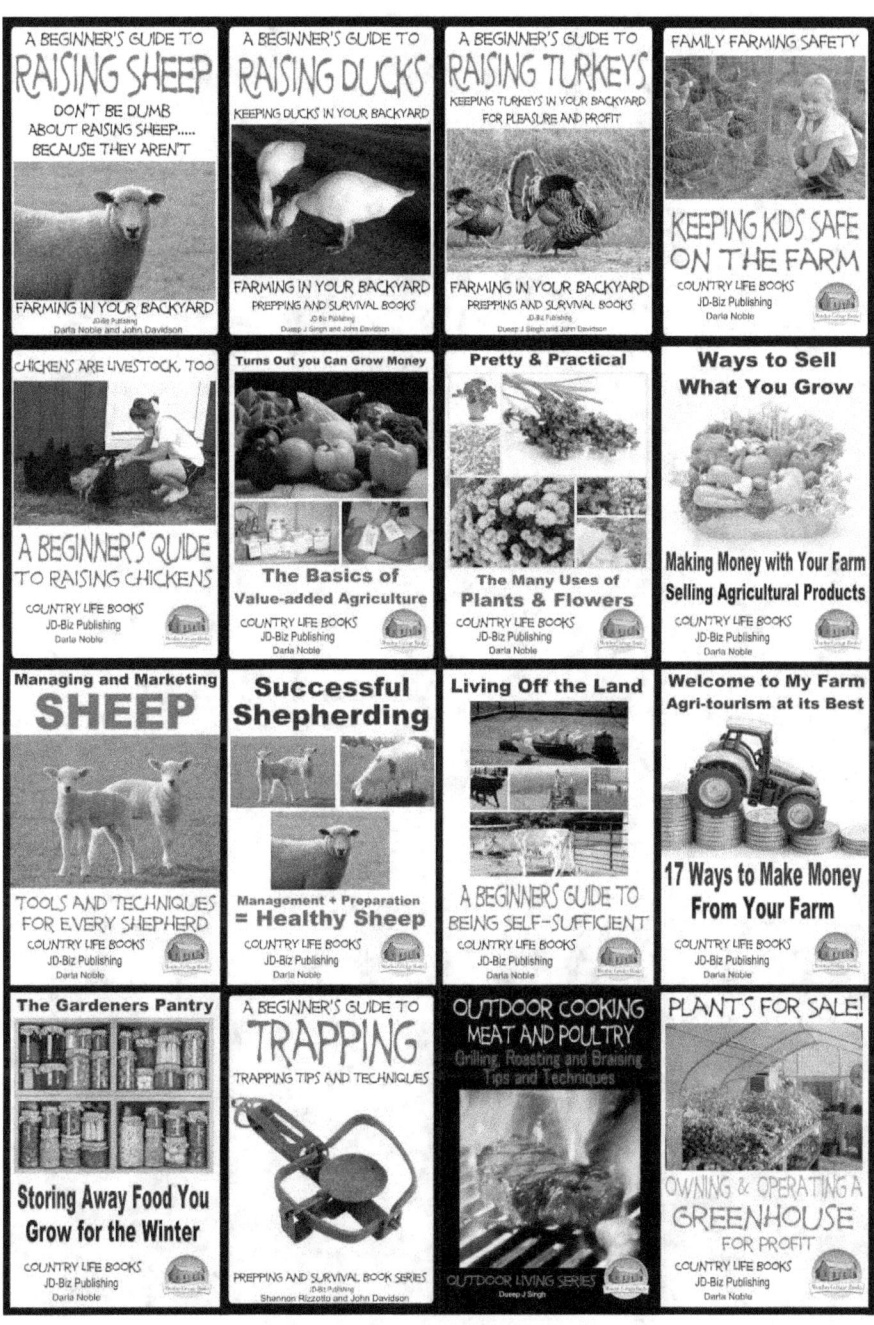

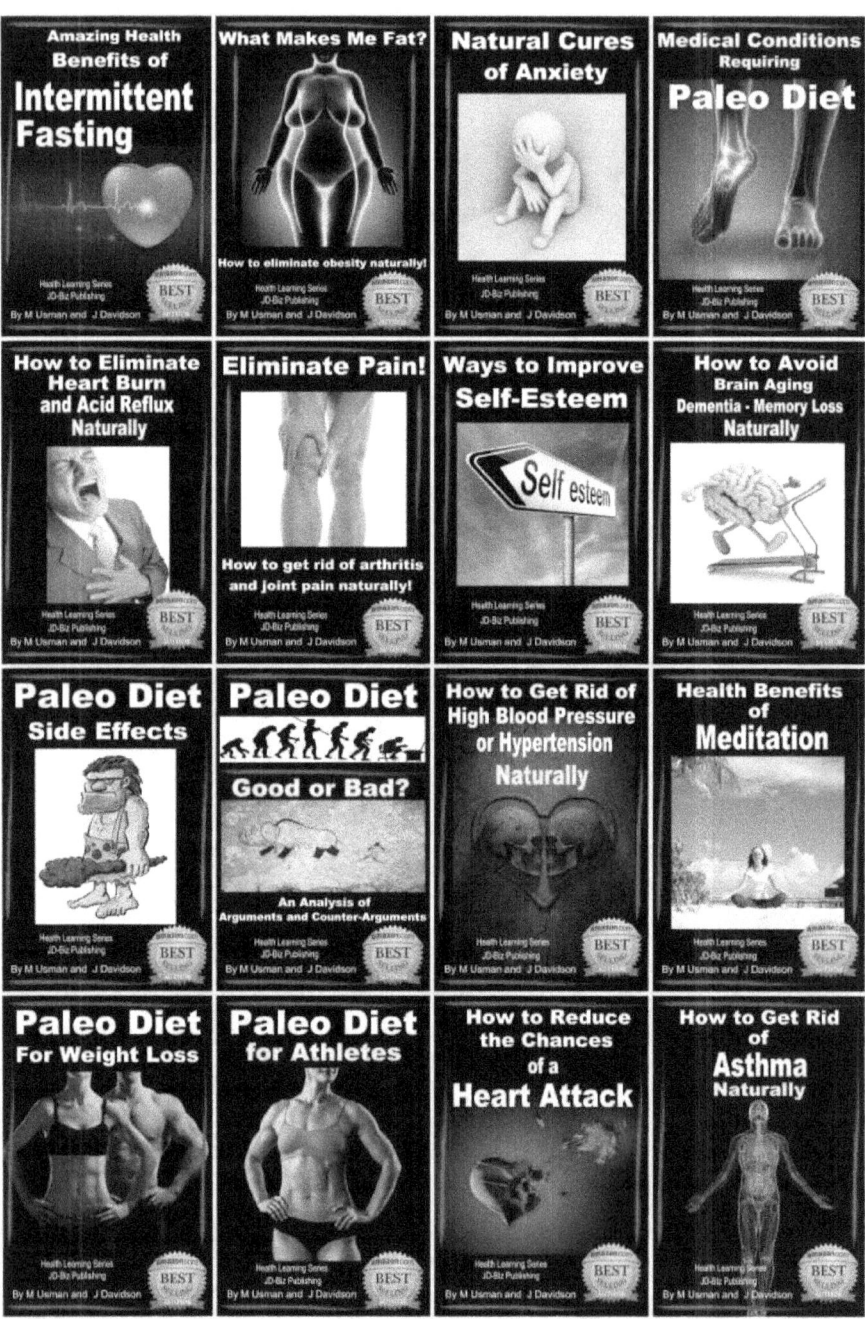

Amazing Animal Book Series

Chinchillas	Beavers	Snakes	Dolphins	Wolves	Walruses
Polar Bears	Turtles	Bees	Frogs	Horses	Monkeys
Dinosaurs	Sharks	Whales	Spiders	Big Cats	Big Mammals of Yellowstone
Animals of Australia	Sasquatch - Yeti Abominable Snowman Bigfoot	Giant Panda Bears	Kittens	Komodo Dragons	Lady Bugs
Animals of North America	Meerkats	Birds of North America	Penguins	Hamsters	Elephants

Learn To Draw Series

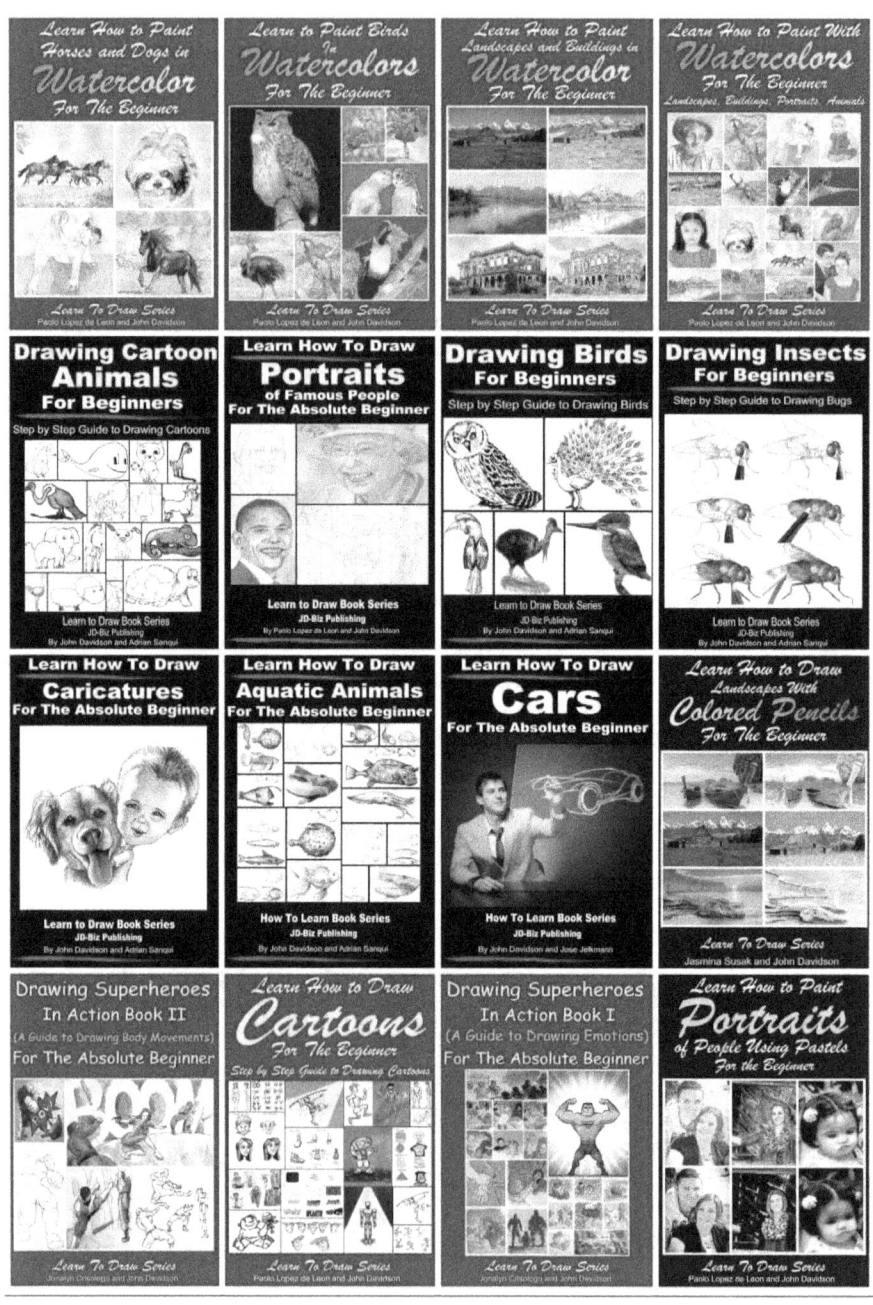

How to Build and Plan Books

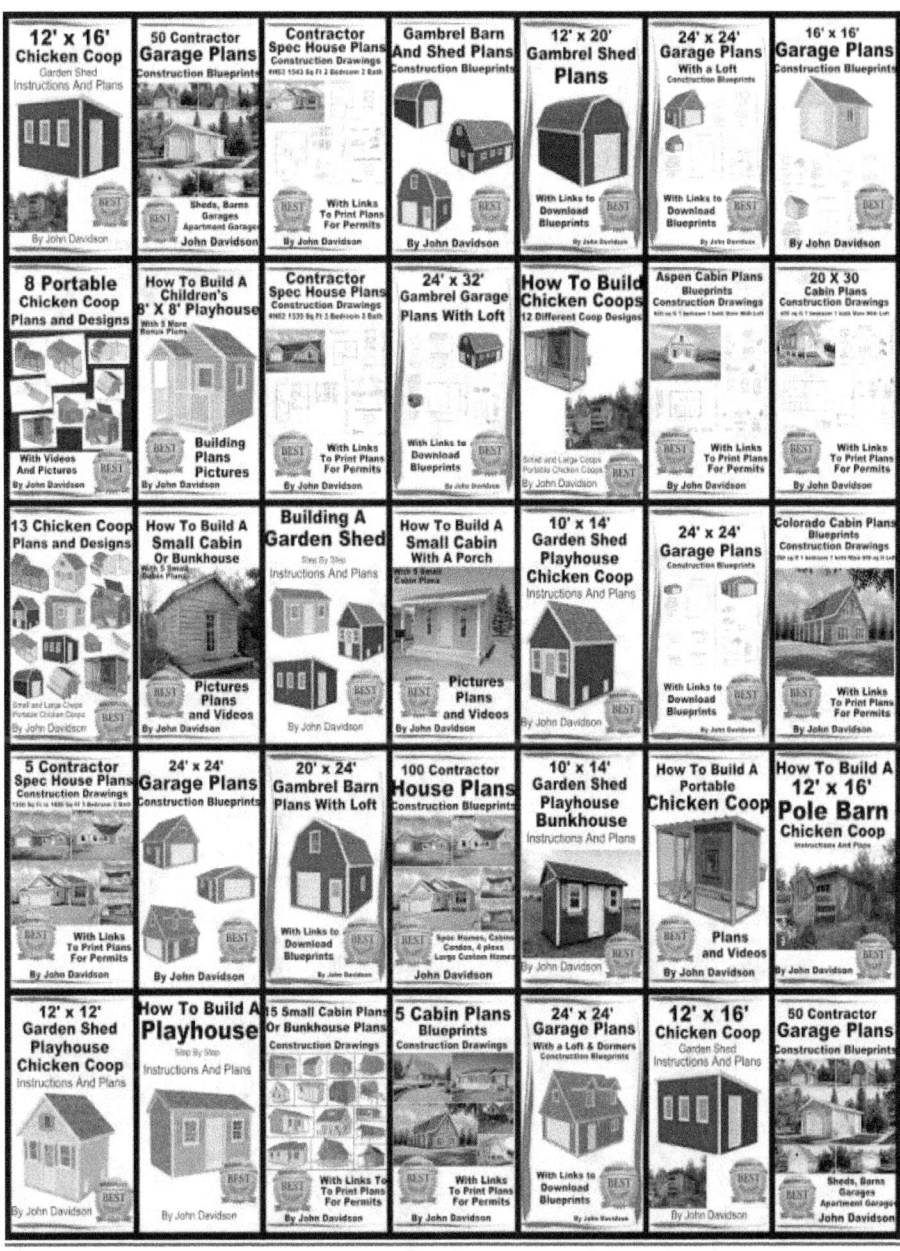

Entrepreneur Book Series

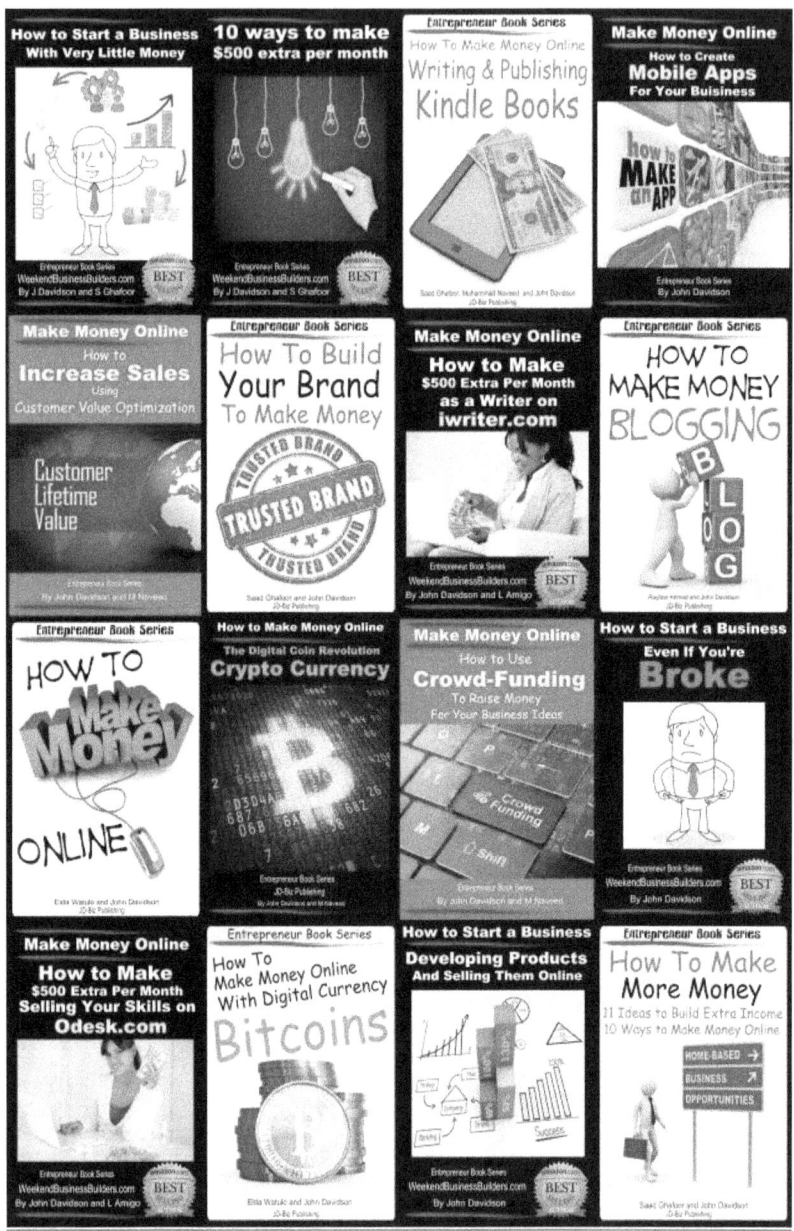

Our books are available at

1. Amazon.com

2. Barnes and Noble

3. Itunes

4. Kobo

5. Smashwords

6. Google Play Books

Publisher

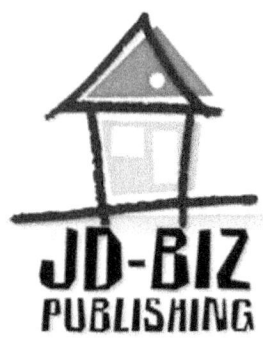

JD-Biz Corp

P O Box 374

Mendon, Utah 84325

http://www.jd-biz.com/

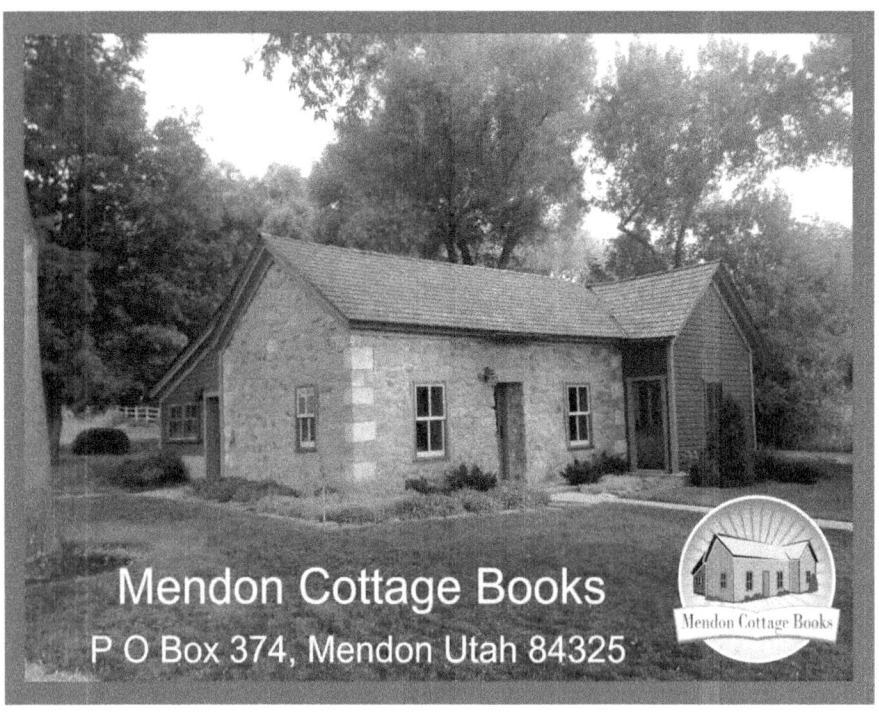

www.ingramcontent.com/pod-product-compliance
Lightning Source LLC
Chambersburg PA
CBHW071145280526
45787CB00003B/1411